Making Your Own Spa at Home

Guide to Create Amazing Spa in Your Home

Copyright © 2020

All rights reserved.

DEDICATION

The author and publisher have provided this e-book to you for your personal use only. You may not make this e-book publicly available in any way. Copyright infringement is against the law. If you believe the copy of this e-book you are reading infringes on the author's copyright, please notify the publisher at: https://us.macmillan.com/piracy

Contents

Get Your Bath To #Bathfluencer Standard 1

The Best Facial Massage Tools For Sculpting And Soothing 32

Get Your Bath To #Bathfluencer Standard

Harness the full power of a good soak by upgrading your bath (simple water doesn't cut it anymore).

Whether you're a fan of fragrant essential oils, bubble bath or a handful of bath salts, the key is in the scent.

'Although aroma is something very personal, and your body will be drawn to what they most need there are specific essential oils that hold properties that will naturally help your mind and body relax. Deeply relaxing oils to look for are naturally sedating vetiver, calming camomile and grounding sandalwood' explains Aromatherapy Associates Global Director of Education and Wellbeing, Christina Salcedas.

Some Bathroom Decor Ideas For You:

Making Your Own Spa at Home

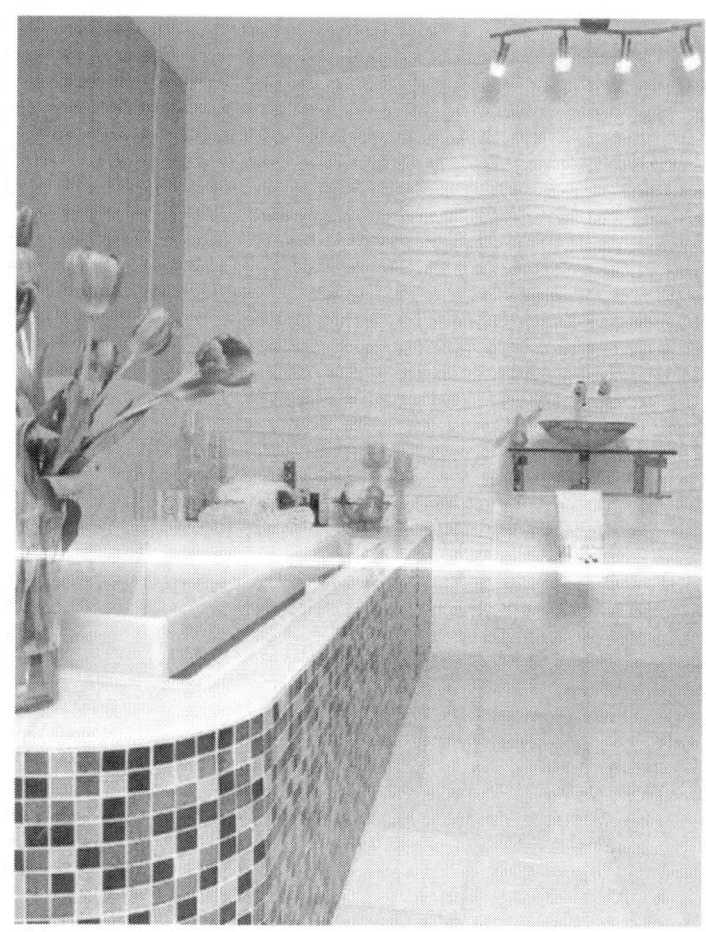

Making Your Own Spa at Home

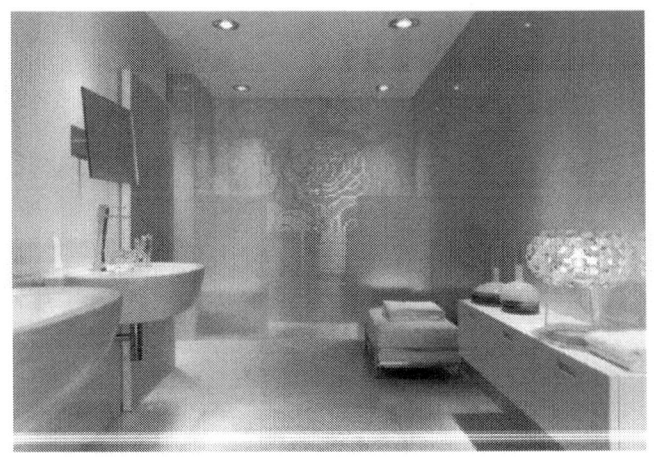

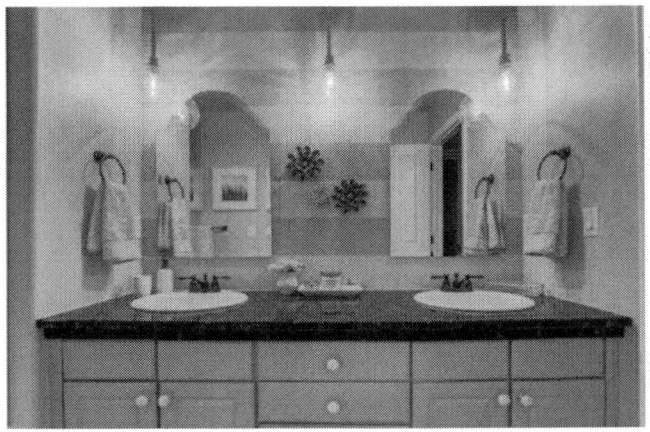

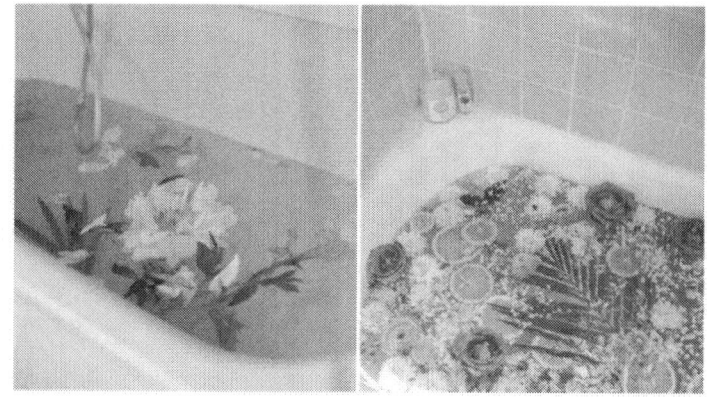
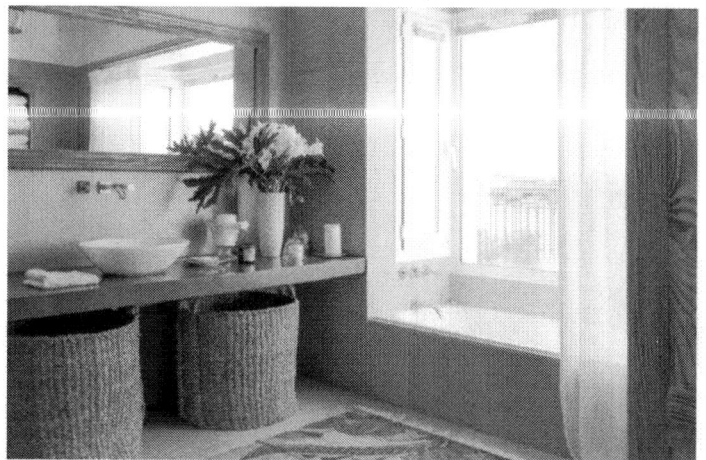

Making Your Own Spa at Home

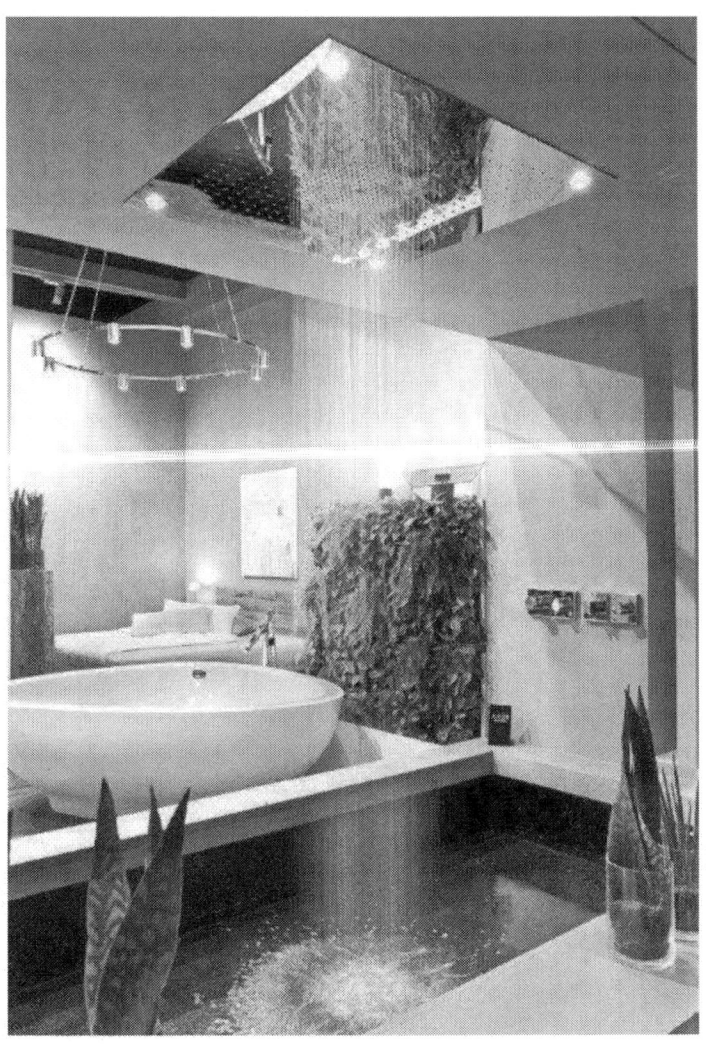

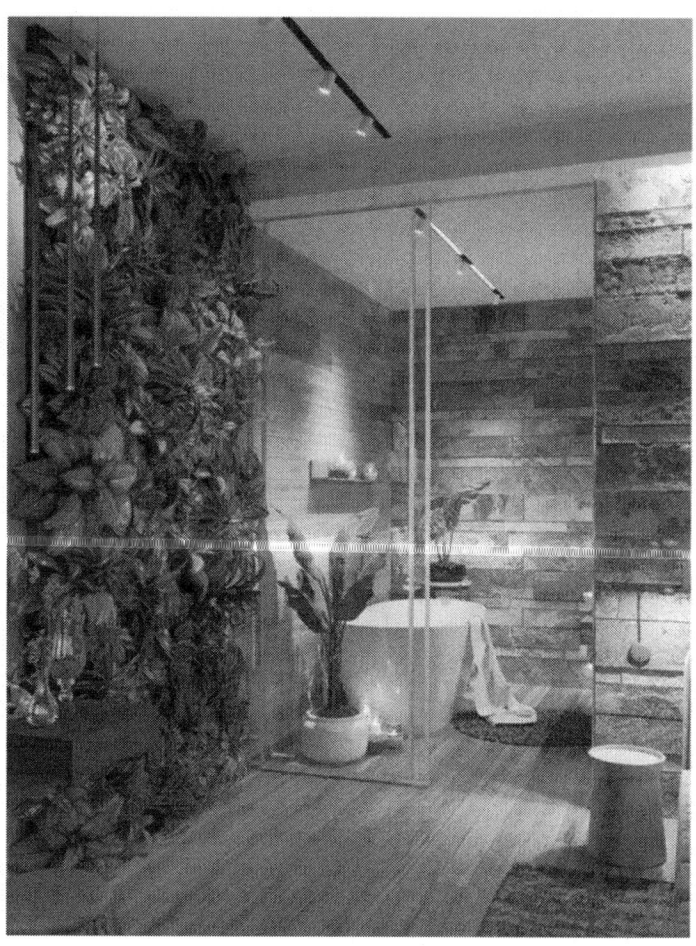

Making Your Own Spa at Home

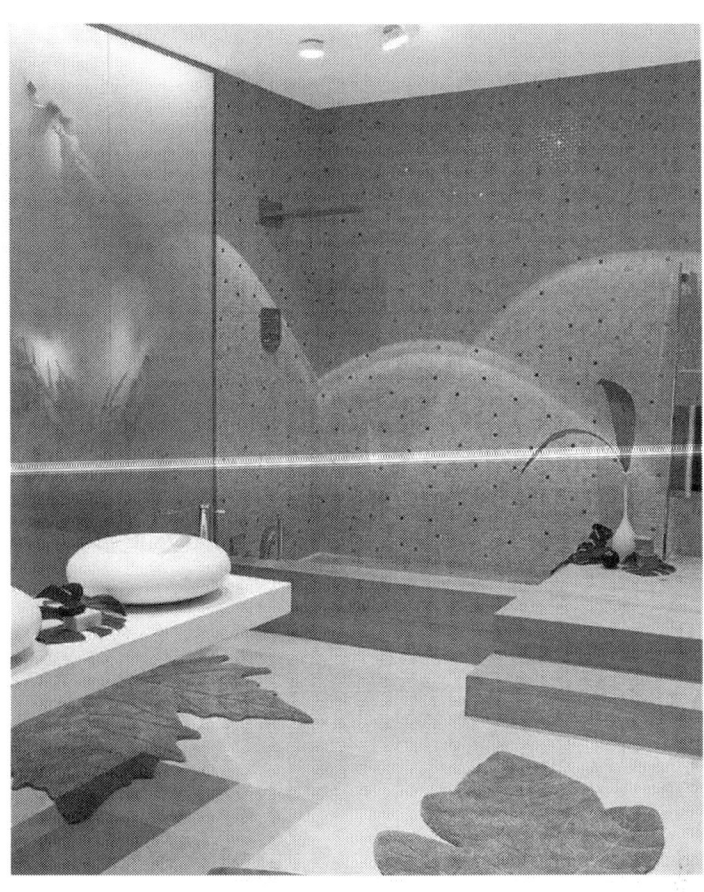

Making Your Own Spa at Home

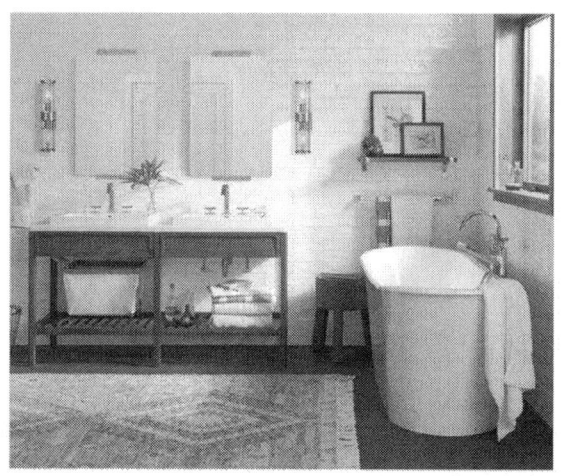

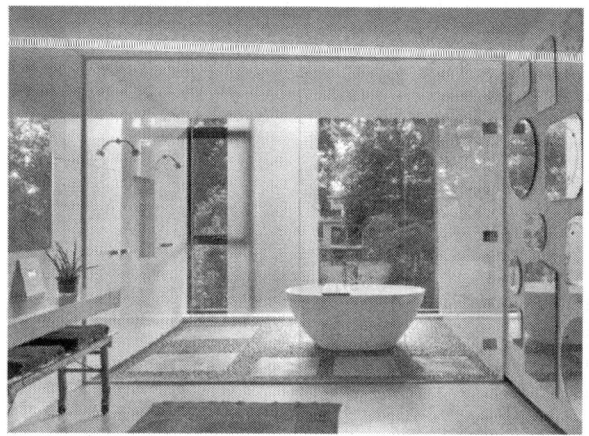

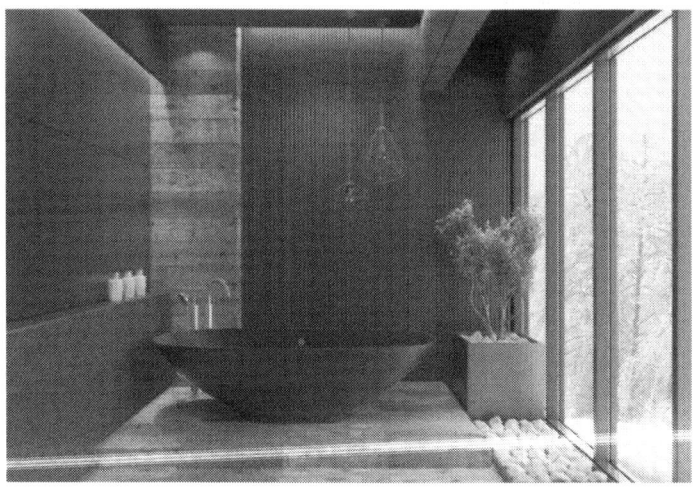

Making Your Own Spa at Home

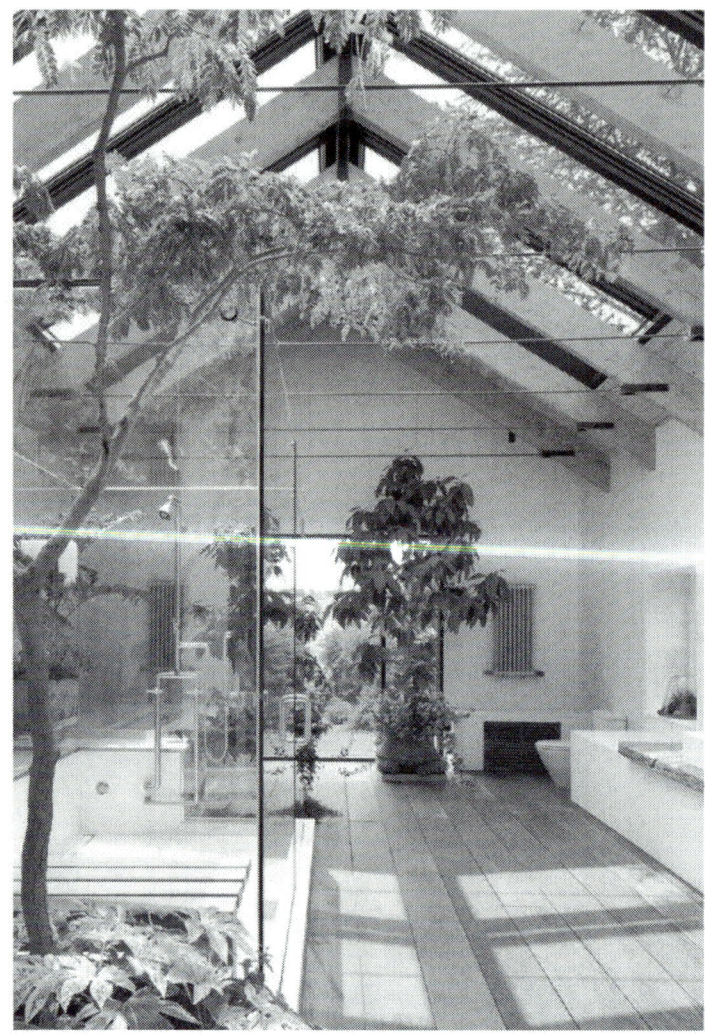

Making Your Own Spa at Home

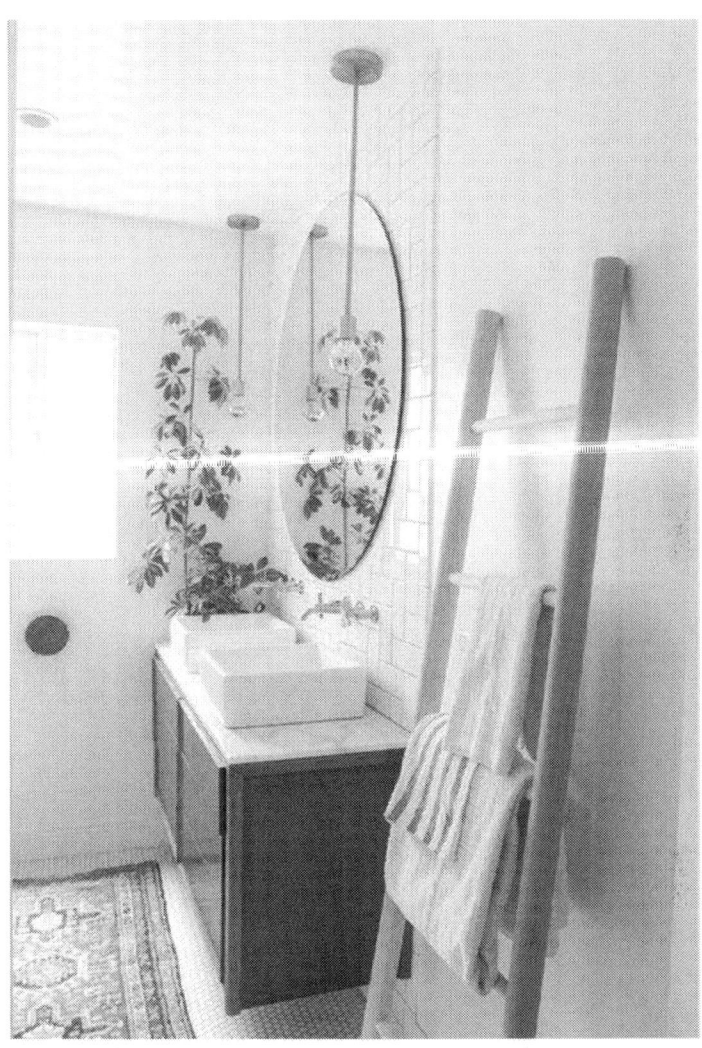

Making Your Own Spa at Home

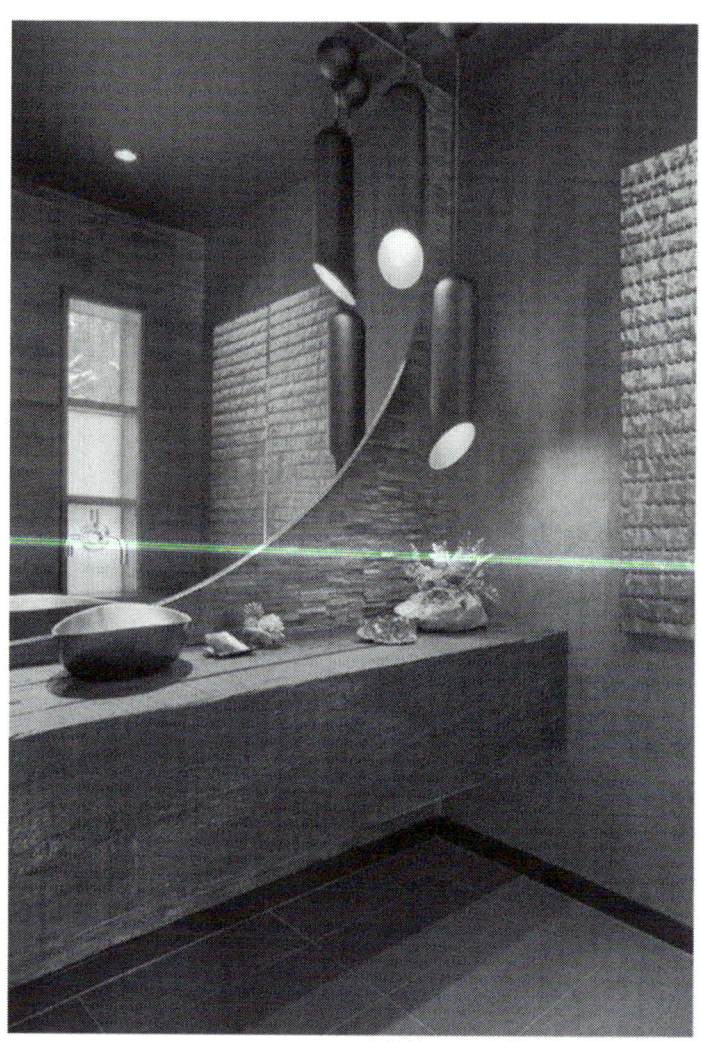

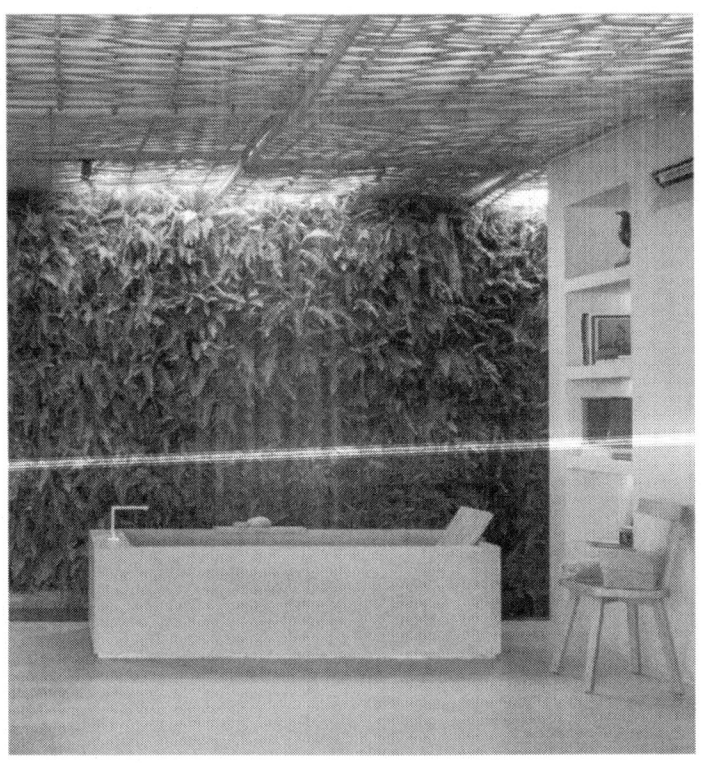

If you're looking for a light relax and don't like scents that are too heavy, Salcedas recommends keeping an eye out for 'Ylang ylang, petigrain and lavender are ideal. If you find your mind is not switching off, or you are still waking in your sleep try things like Frankincense or Camomile.'

There's also a lot of science behind the relaxing qualities of a bath too. 'Bathing is proven to lower the stress hormone, cortisol and stimulates the release of endorphins. There are also studies that show bathing can lower blood pressure to support heart health too', explains Salcedas.

Don't have a bath? No problem. Apply your body oil right before stepping in the shower, the hot water and steam will create a relaxing sauna effect and allow you to breath in all the relaxing scent benefits.

Clear Your Mind

It's easier said than done but technology has been a huge helping hand in getting our brains to switch off so we can finally relax.

Meditation apps are all the craze (ELLE love Headspace and Calm) to help switch off any last minute work thoughts or worries.

This content is imported from {embed-name}. You may be able to find the same content in another format, or you may be able to find more information, at their web site.

If you want an offline method (because who needs blue light right before bed), Salcedas reveals her simple breathing trick:

'I am a real advocate of simple breathing routines, so you don't have to think too much about what you are doing and really do it well. Box breathing is a great example of that. Breathing in for four seconds, hold for four seconds, then breathe out for four seconds and hold the breath out for four… and repeat at least you got it… four times'.

Light A Candle

There's no denying the peace that comes with lighting a fresh candle. Part of the relaxing quality of a spa is the scent that envelopes you as soon as you step foot in it and your house should be no different.

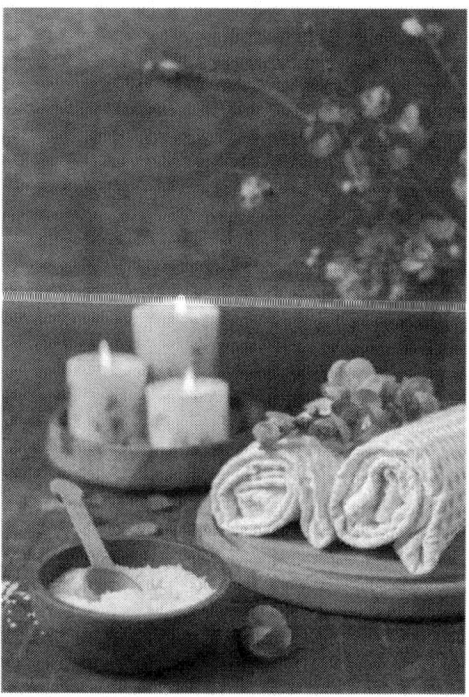

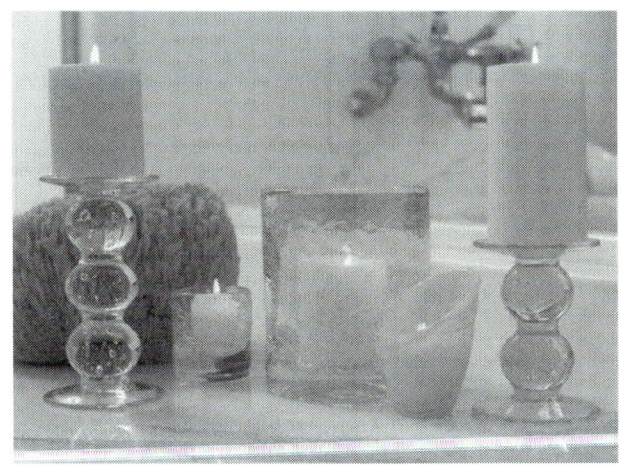

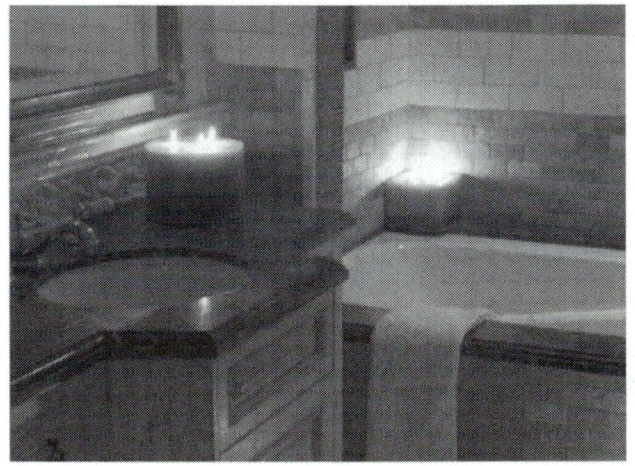

Making Your Own Spa at Home

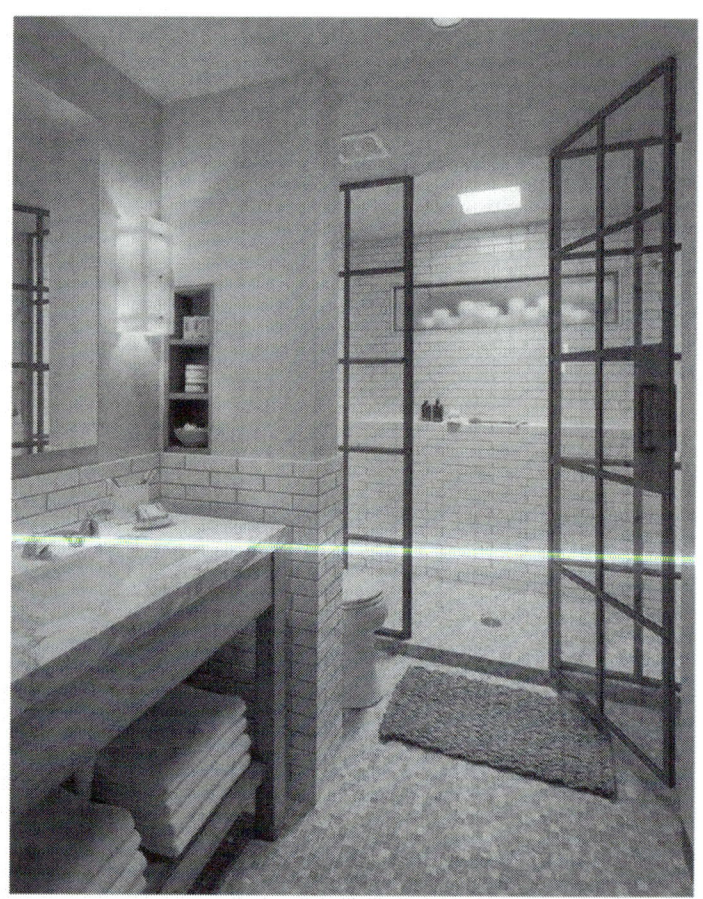

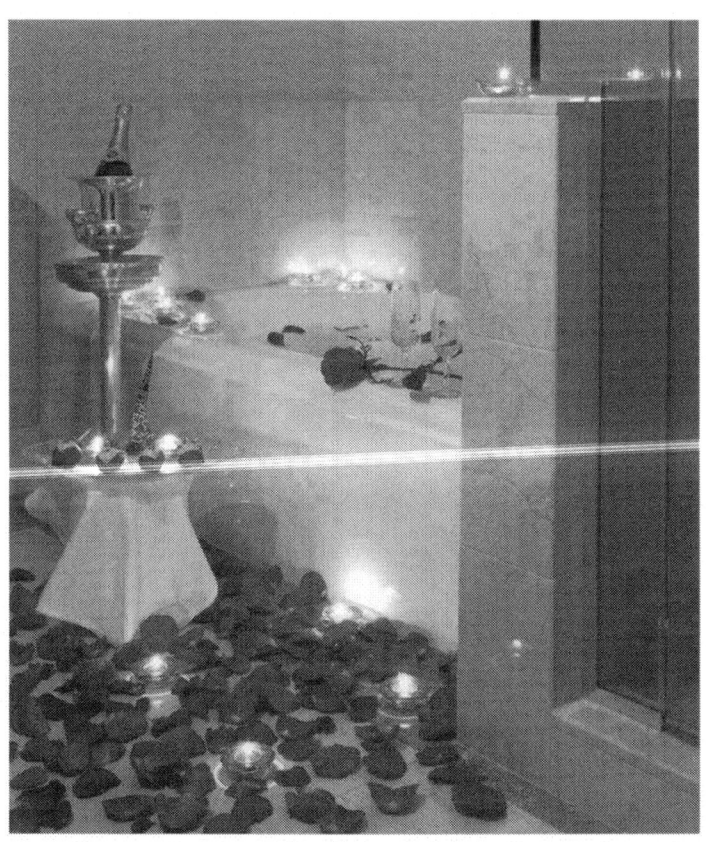

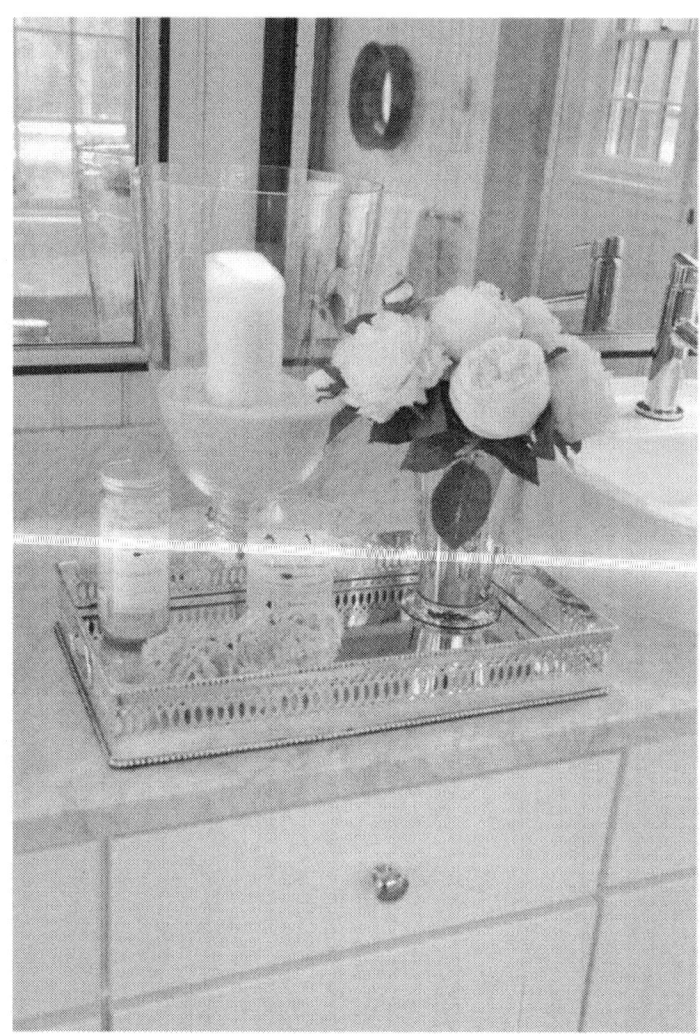

Making Your Own Spa at Home

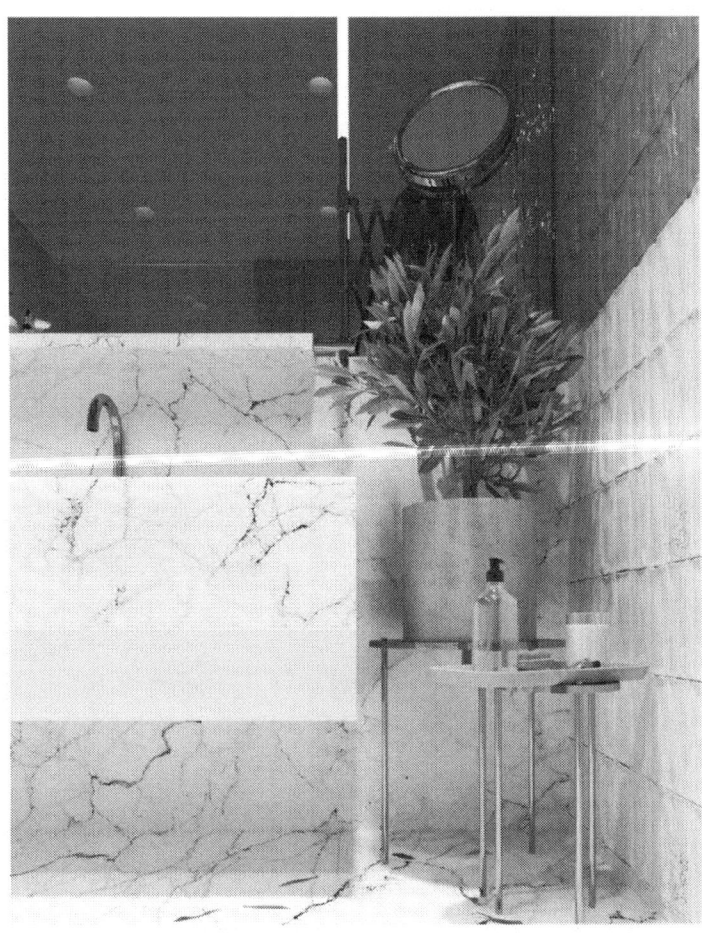

As with essential oils, if you want a relaxing scent, go for candles with notes of lavender, camomile or sandalwood to help you drift off to sleep right before bed.

If you're not a fan of candles, try a calming pillow spray or room spray to do the trick.

Some Candle Safety Tips

Keep Candles Where You Can See Them

This is something I am particularly aware of now that I am a mother. I never leave my candles unattended, out of sight, or in a high traffic area of the house where a child or a pet could easily knock them over.

For me, candles can bring such a sense of relaxation. They are like a little piece of a holiday that can just drain the stress of a busy day away, but it is important to never fall asleep when a candle is burning. I can understand the temptation — believe me, but it just isn't worth the risk. If you are having trouble falling asleep, use a lava lamp. It's a lot safer!

Keep Them Away From Children And Pets

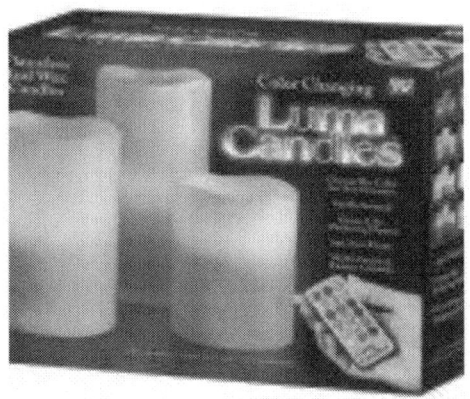

Our children love to imitate us. If we love something, they are automatically attracted to it. That means keeping your candles, matches or lighters in a safe place when they are not in use and teaching kids that real candles are not toys.

I know how much my son likes them, so I have given him battery operated ones of his own. They aren't as nice as real candles, obviously, but he can use them whenever he wants. The little, electric tea-lights that you can find in dollar and discount stores make great stocking stuffers, and they actually teach children not to leave candles lit when they aren't around to enjoy them because the batteries will go dead.

It's actually the cutest thing. My son is very empathetic, and he likes to surprise me with a candle lit snack or an offer to cuddle up together with popcorn and a movie with a pair of his electric candles. It's his way of keeping Mommy happy and creating the perfect atmosphere for a happy home. Is that training for the future or what! Candle purists might think I'm crazy, but they've actually become something that is an important part of our family life.

Choose A Safe Location

Curtains are also something to keep in mind when choosing a location to burn your candles and any other flowing or portable textiles, like blankets, bedding, flammable party decorations or towels. I love to have a candle-lit bath, sweet milk bubbles up to my chin, the works, but candles and towels do not mix!

Curtains can blow around in the breeze of an open window, so you can't forget about any objects or other factors that might move into the danger zone. Be aware of any drafts or air currents, vents or fans.

Candles can also mark some areas, just because their container can get hot, especially as the candle burns down. In fact, it's suggested that you never burn a candle right down to the end, for just that reason. Getting some cheap, nonflammable coasters are a good idea, and if they get wax on them, you can always throw them out. It's always possible that the heat can cause what they're sitting on to burst into flame as well, so don't use a book instead, and make sure they are somewhere stable that won't get knocked down.

Use A Good Container Or Holder & Trim Your Wick

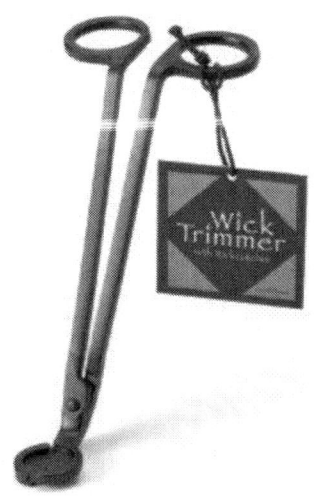

Maybe it isn't always a safety issue, but wax is something else to consider. It can easily stain fabric or other surfaces. That's more of a worry with candlesticks, obviously, than votives. That's one of the reasons why I prefer candles that burn into a container. There is less mess and everything is more controllable. They aren't perfectly safe, but there is a bit of a shield there when it comes to pets and kids. Don't use candles with wooden or plastic holders that can catch fire or that have flammable decorations like ribbons or tree-bark.

Remembering to trim your wick to 5-7 mm or 1/4 inch before you light it can also make a big difference, and do it after that every 2-3 hours to prevent the flame getting too big. Extinguishing it with a snuffer cuts down on wax splatters too and don't even think about putting it out with water if it's in a glass container. That can be really dangerous and cause the glass to shatter.

Think Safety First

Every day is special enough to deserve candles in my house. I don't know about you, but they always put a smile on my face. If you always keep in mind that they can also be dangerous, and you follow common sense and safe practices, then they will always put a smile on your face too.

Treat Yourself To A Facial Massage

Facials that actually improve your skin sometimes shouldn't be the most comfortable (no one said extraction was ever easy) but facial massaging meets in the middle to give you a sculpted effect without pummelling your face.

'The practice of facial exercise has a long history but it's often news to people that over 40 muscles make up the scaffolding of the face. And just like the muscles in the body, the more you move them, the more lifted, tightened and tone they become', explains Inge Theron, Founder of FaceGym.

This content is imported from Instagram. You may be able to find the same content in another format, or you may be able to find more information, at their web site.

Theron breaks down the three techniques you can use to get that sculpted effect:

1. Chin Press Up X 3

'Make a V with our hand and rest your chin in the V. Pull your lips over your top teeth hold for 5 seconds and repeat (do this 10 times). Move the hand to either side of the chin with the length of your fingers covering your ears, and make the sound Eeeee with your mouth x 10. Put your ring fingers inside your mouth on either side, pull the skin to the side and use your jaw muscles to bring the fingers back in to touch your teeth x 10'

2. Fish Pose

'Hold your collarbone with your hands on either side, tilt your head back slowly till you feel a stretch and then start opening and closing your mouth like a fish making circles as if you were saying "ouch"'.

3. Eeeek

'Still holding your hands on your collarbone, look ahead and say eeeeeeek x 10 times'.

If you also find you grind your teeth at night without realising, releasing that tension built up in your jaw can really help you get to sleep and minimise any teeth-grinding-induced headaches.

If you don't have the upper body strength, there are a range of at-home skincare tools that can do all the heavy lifting for you to work out those tight knots.

The Best Facial Massage Tools For Sculpting And Soothing

They might feel heavenly on a tight jawline, but the best face massagers out there will do so much more than soothe the day's stresses (which, right now, are plentiful). From aiding lymphatic drainage to increasing your skin's ability to soak up a serum, there are so many reasons to invest in a stone, roller, or tech-powered device.

While every skin type can use a face massage tool, deciding which one to invest in can be tricky – today, the options are plentiful.

One end of the spectrum is rooted in tradition. The ubiquitous jade roller – as well as its gua-sha sister – has beginnings in ancient

Eastern medicine, used to cool skin, soothe overworked muscles and even shift energy blockages in the body.

If ancient wisdom feels a little at odds with your boundary-pushing skincare routine, consider the wealth of high-tech options. Now, advanced technology is taking face massage tools to new heights, incorporating sonic vibrations, gold-plated metal and even microcurrents to stimulate the skin. Used consistently, these devices can lead to more pronounced cheekbones, a tighter jawline, and reduced wrinkles. In the case of vibrational tools, research has even indicated an increase in the skin's absorption of topical products.

Here, discover the *Bazaar* team's verdict on the best face massage tools to try now.

1. The Drug Store

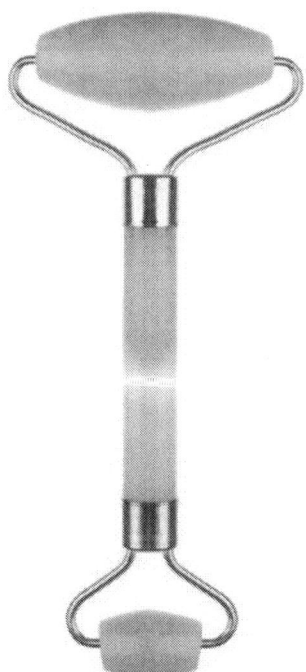

Jade Face Roller

£19.99

Thedrug.store

Crafted from pure green jade, The Drug Store's roller is the perfect entry route into facial massage. The rounded stone tips are designed to feel comfortable in the smaller contours of your face, while the fresh-from-the-fridge stone will instantly cool and de-puff. Roll it upwards and outwards over a favourite serum to increase circulation and shift underlying fluid.

2.   **Mount Lai**

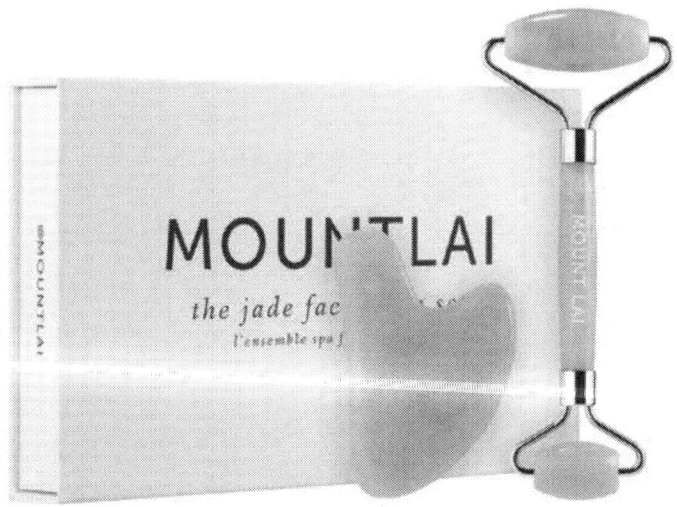

The Jade Facial Spa Set

£44

Beautybay.com

This sleek set contains both a double-ended jade roller and a matching gua-sha tool, so you can mix and match depending on your mood. It'll make a thoughtful gift, too.

3.   **Odacité**

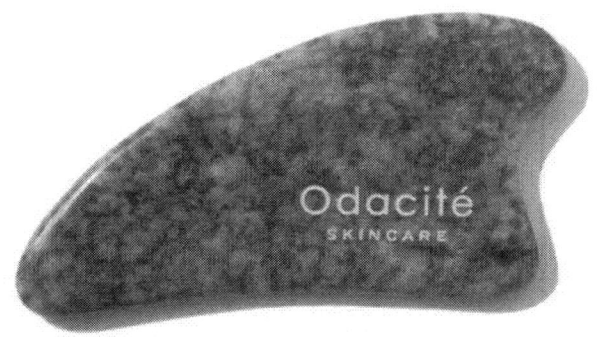

Gua Sha Blue Sodalite Beauty Tool

£40

Spacenk.com

It might be a thing of beauty, but Odacité's blue sodalite massage tool is coveted for more than just its good looks. This perfectly smooth tool is shaped for a serious gua-sha massage: use the wide lengths to smooth and de-puff, and the double-pronged end to sculpt a sharper jawline.

4. Sarah Champan

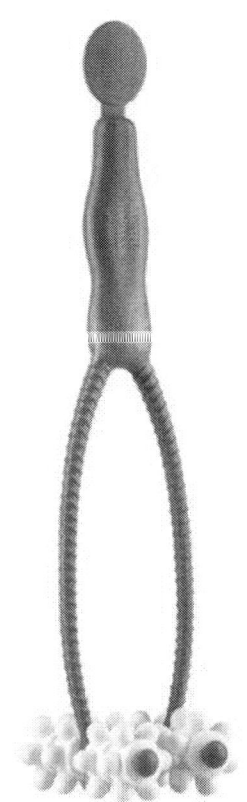

The Facialift

£3

Cultbeauty.co.uk

Fans of Sarah Chapman's treatments should snap this one up immediately – it's designed to mimic the facialist's signature kneading massage technique. Simple yet effective (and surprisingly easy to use), the rotating massagers run up from the chin to the ears, aiding lymphatic drainage. With toxins swept swiftly away, puffiness is diminished and breakouts prevented.

5. MODM

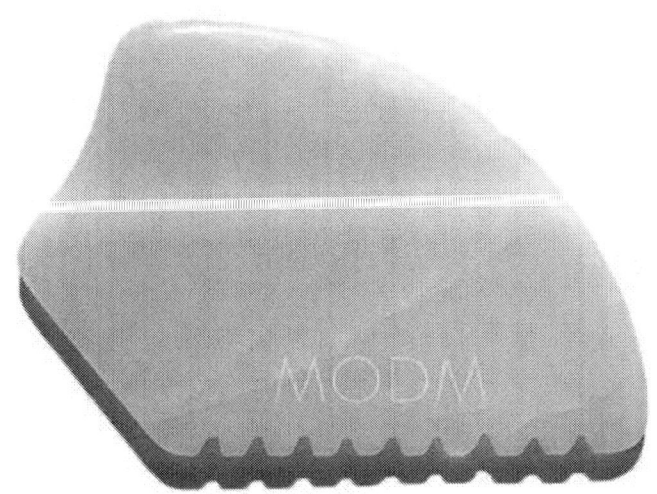

Gua Sha Face Tool

£26

Thedrug.store

A gua sha may be new to our beauty arsenal, but they've been integral to ancient Eastern routines for centuries. Used in 'skin scraping' therapies, these smoothly contoured stones are believed to direct energy, release blockages and boost the lymphatic system.

Run Modm's pure rose quartz iteration over serum-soaked skin to release blockages that can lead to puffiness and breakouts. Regular use will reveal strikingly sharp cheekbones.

The technique might be trickier to master than a jade roller, but it also offers more precision — ideal for anyone looking to target a specific area.

6. **Angela Caglia**

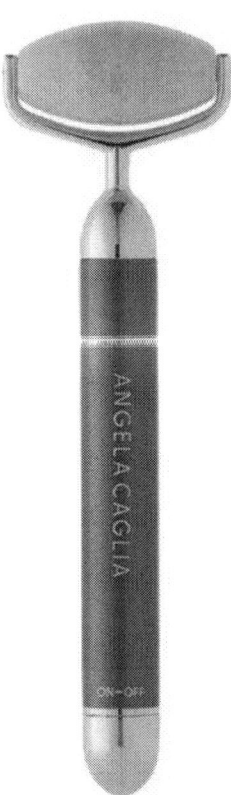

Vibrating Rose Quartz Face Sculpting Roller

£154

Net-a-porter.com

As seen in Courtney Cox's grasp in one of the year's most puzzling paparazzi shots, (the actress was rolling her complexion during a dinner), Angela Caglia's vibrational massager is clearly the A-list tool of choice.

A cut above traditional designs, this advanced wand uses sonic vibrations – over 6000 per minute – to lift and tone the skin in an instant.

Moisturise, Then Moisturise Again

No one has ever left a spa with dry skin and if you have, you're not doing it right. Skin that's parched often feels uncomfortable and tight, which is not the aim of the game.

Stressed out skin often results in angry skin. We're talking flare ups in skin conditions such as rosacea and eczema and will often result in some very unwanted pimples.

Stick to a moisturising routine (that includes the body too) to help get you to your best skin ever, which in turn, will boost happiness.

10 Best Natural Moisturizers For Dry Skin

1. DIY Shea Butter Homemade Face Moisturizer For Dry Skin

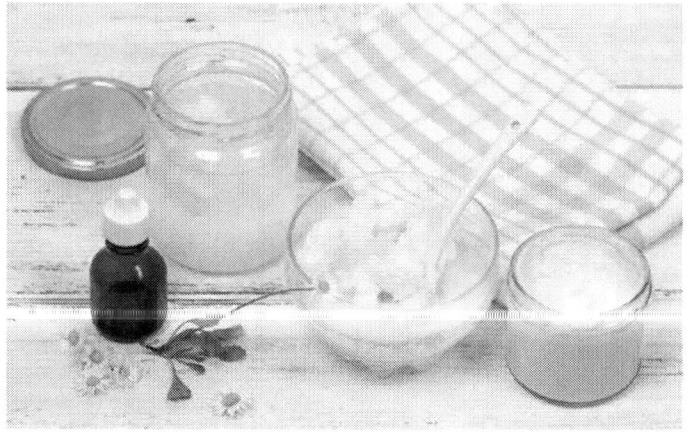

You Will Need

- ½ cup shea butter
- 6-7 drops sea buckthorn oil
- 6-7 drops rosehip seed oil

- 6-7 drops geranium oil
- 1 teaspoon avocado oil

Method

- Melt the shea butter in a double boiler**.
- Once it has softened, remove it from the heat.
- Add avocado oil and mix.
- Add the essential oils and whip the mixture well until it develops a creamy texture.
- Store it in a glass jar and use it as your daily face cream.

Why This Works

Sea buckthorn oil is extremely effective in treating eczema and soothes dry and itchy skin. Rosehip seed, geranium, and avocado oils have an equally soothing effect on your dry skin while shea butter keeps it moisturized and nourished.

To make a double boiler, pour some water in a saucepan and place it on the stove. Place a heat-proof glass container that fits snugly over the saucepan. Once the water starts simmering, keep the butter on the glass container and let it melt. Keep stirring until it melts.

2. Natural Face Moisturizer For Dry Skin

You Will Need

- ½ cup argan oil (you can also take jojoba oil or hempseed oil)
- ½ teaspoon emu oil
- 4-6 drops essential oil (lemongrass, rose geranium, rose, chamomile, palmarosa, rosemary, lavender, or peppermint)

Method

1. Take a glass bottle and pour argan oil into it.
2. Add the other oils to the argan oil and mix well.
3. Use the blend to massage your skin.

Why This Works

Argan oil is light and suitable for soothing dry skin. Emu oil is a natural emollient that helps in locking moisture in your skin and heals it from within. Essential oils (the listed ones) have an overall healing effect, especially for dry and sensitive skin.

3. Beeswax Moisturizer For Dry Skin

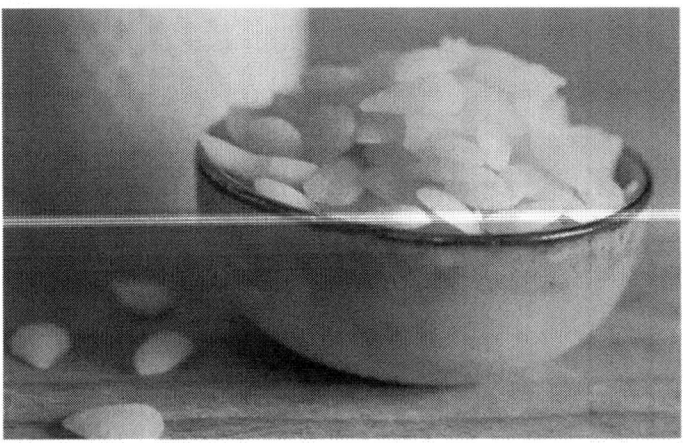

You Will Need

- ¼ cup beeswax pellets
- ½ cup coconut oil
- ½ cup olive oil

- 10 drops essential oil (patchouli, Roman chamomile, vanilla, sandalwood, frankincense, clary sage, lavender, or geranium oil)

Method

1. Use a double boiler to melt the beeswax.
2. Once it melts, remove it from the boiler and let it cool.
3. Add the coconut and olive oils and whip well.
4. Add the essential oil(s).
5. Whip the mixture well until you get a creamy texture.
6. Transfer the mixture to a glass jar and store it in a cool and dry place (do not refrigerate).

Why This Works

Both beeswax and olive oil heal skin conditions such as atopic dermatitis (eczema). Coconut oil provides added moisturization to your skin, and essential oils promote further healing.

4. Gentle Aloe Vera Moisturizer For Dry Skin

You Will Need

- 1 cup aloe vera gel (use store-bought gel or scoop out the gel from an aloe leaf)
- 12 tablespoons beeswax
- ¼ cup coconut oil
- ¼ cup almond oil
- 10 drops essential oil(s) (pick any from the oils mentioned in the above recipes)

Method

1. Melt the beeswax, coconut, and almond oils in a double boiler.
2. Pour the oils into a blender and let the mixture cool down.
3. Add the essential oils and the aloe vera gel. Blend until you get a creamy texture.

4. Store the mixture a glass jar. You can even store it in the refrigerator.

Why This Works

Aloe vera soothes your skin and reduces inflammation (itches and dry patches). Beeswax heals your skin and keeps it moisturized, and essential oils prevent infection and help in healing your skin.

5. DIY Nourishing Face And Body Cream For Dry Skin

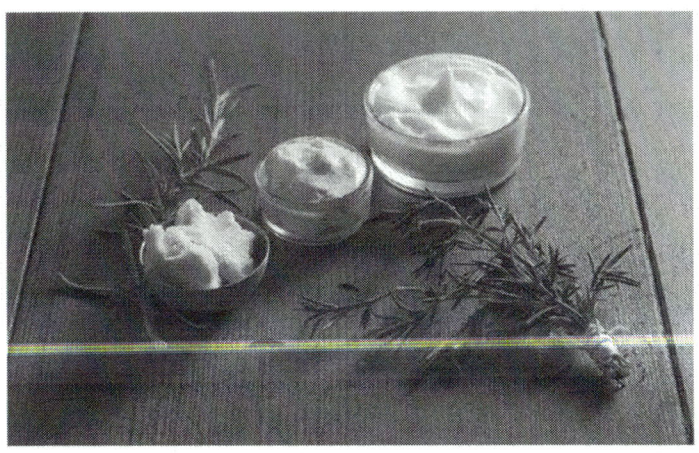

You Will Need

- ½ cup shea butter
- 2 tablespoons almond oil
- 5 drops rosemary essential oil
- 10 drops lavender essential oil
- 3 drops tea tree essential oil

- 3 drops carrot seed essential oil

Method

1. Melt the shea butter in a double boiler. Add almond oil after it melts and turn the burner off.

2. Let the mixture cool (but do not let it solidify) and then add the essential oils.

3. Whip the mixture well. You can use a whisker or blend it in a mixer (for a few seconds).

4. Scoop out the creamy mixture into a glass jar. Store it at room temperature.

5. Massage the cream on your body and face.

Why This Works

The essential oils protect your skin cells. All these oils have antiseptic properties that heal infections and prevent skin damage and rashes caused by excessive dryness. Shea butter and almond oil keep your skin moisturized and nourished.

6. DIY Honey And Glycerin Moisturizer For Dry Skin

You Will Need

- 1 teaspoon honey
- 2 teaspoons glycerin
- 1 teaspoon lemon juice (diluted)
- 2 teaspoons green tea

Method

1. Mix all the ingredients well.
2. Massage the mixture gently on your skin for a few minutes.
3. Leave it on overnight.
4. Wash it off the next day.

Why This Works

Glycerin and honey are humectants that keep your skin moisturized and hydrated. Lemon brightens up your skin while the green tea calms your skin and keeps infection at bay.

Note: Lemon juice may not suit everyone, so do a patch test first. You can skip adding lemon juice altogether if you want to.

7. Natural Face Moisturizer For Dry Skin

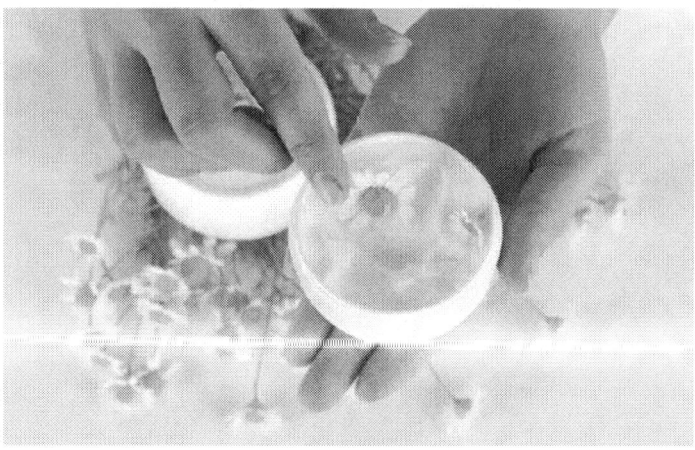

You Will Need

- 1 teaspoon chamomile tea (or dried chamomile flowers)
- ½ cup water
- 1 tablespoon lanolin

- 1 tablespoon beeswax
- ½ cup sweet almond oil
- 1 vitamin A capsule
- 1 vitamin E capsule
- 3 drops geranium essential oil

Method

1. Put the chamomile tea (or flowers) in the water, simmer for 10 minutes and strain the liquid.

2. Melt the lanolin (if you are not using liquid lanolin) and beeswax in a double boiler.

3. Let the mixture cool down. Add the chamomile brew.

4. Pierce the vitamin capsules and squeeze the liquid into the mixture. Keep stirring and then add the essential oil.

5. Whip it well until you get a creamy texture.

6. Transfer the mixture to a glass jar and store it in a cool and dark place.

7. Massage on your body and face as and when required.

Why This Works

This homemade cream provides intense hydration to your skin. Chamomile has anti-inflammatory properties that have a softening and soothing effect on irritated skin. Almond oil and beeswax provide nourishment to your skin and prevent drying.

8. Nourishing Day Cream For Dry Skin

You Will Need

- 3 tablespoons sweet almond oil
- 1 tablespoon avocado oil
- 3 teaspoon beeswax
- 2 drops lavender essential oil
- 2 tablespoons mineral water

- 1 drop peppermint essential oil

Method

1. Melt the beeswax and the oils in a double boiler.

2. Warm the mineral water (don't boil) and slowly add it to the molten beeswax and oil mix. Keep stirring.

3. Remove the beeswax from the heat once it melts and let it cool down.

4. Add the essential oils and whip vigorously.

5. Scoop out the cream into a glass jar and store it in a cool, dry place.

6. Use it as a day cream.

Why This Works

Avocado and almond oils contain UV filters that protect your skin from the harmful UV rays while keeping it moisturized. The essential oils (lavender and peppermint) also have a sun protection factor.

These oils protect your skin from UV rays and keep your skin healthy.

9. DIY Gentle And Hydrating Moisturizer For Dry Skin

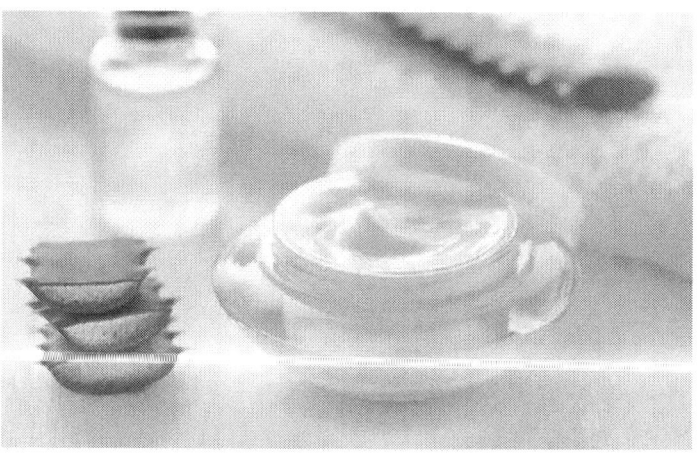

You Will Need

- 3 tablespoons shea butter
- 1 teaspoon vitamin E oil
- 1 teaspoon aloe vera gel
- 3 tablespoons apricot seed oil

- 5 drops helichrysum essential oil
- 5 drops of myrrh essential oil
- 3 drops clary sage essential oil

Method

1. Melt the shea butter in a double boiler and allow it to cool down a bit.

2. Whisk the butter once it cools down and add the oils and aloe vera gel. Keep mixing.

3. Once it reaches a creamy consistency, transfer the cream to a glass container.

4. Apply it to your face and body as and when required.

Why This Works

Shea butter has amazing healing and moisturizing properties. It contains vitamins A, D, and E that keep your skin nourished and help in healing eczema and other dry skin issues. Apricot seed oil goes along well with shea butter as it is non-irritant, and just like shea butter, it keeps your skin moisturized.

10. Revitalizing Hibiscus Moisturizer For Dry Skin

You Will Need

- 2 tablespoons hibiscus tea
- 1 cup extra virgin coconut oil

Method

1. Grind the hibiscus tea into powder.
2. Melt the coconut oil in a double boiler.
3. Add the hibiscus tea powder to the oil and cover it for a while.
4. Use a cheesecloth to strain the oil and separate the tea from the oil.
5. Let the oil cool down until it solidifies.
6. Whip it well in a mixer for about a minute or two.
7. Transfer the pinkish cream to a glass jar and apply to your skin.

Why This Works

In Africa, hibiscus pulp is often used for wound healing and soothing the skin. It contains anthocyanins and antioxidants that enhance skin health. Coconut oil has a calming and soothing impact on your skin and also keeps it moisturized.

A Mask A Week, Keeps The Split Ends At Bay

We often blow off a hair mask due to time restrictions but we should be embracing the time they take to sink in. Not only will your hair thank you for it but it will also give your mind some time to switch off too. Apply a mask, grab a book and relax.

Add a mask into your weekly hair ritual to really reap the benefits. Naeemah LaFond, Global Artistic Director for Cult US haircare brand amika believes that a 'weekly deep conditioning is essential to beautiful healthy hair. To avoid tangling and to really feel the effects of the massage it's best not to gather all of your hair into your hands to massage. Let the hair hang and use your fingertips to massage the roots thoroughly.'

There's a mask for every hair concern, whether you have coloured hair and want to enhance the colour, or have straw-like dry ends and want to add a hit of moisture, there's a mask out there for you.

Have A Clear Out

In true Marie Kondo style, nothing is more stressful than a messy and over-cluttered home. When was the last time you went into a messy spa? Hopefully never.

'I always stress the importance of creating the environment first and foremost. Declutter, tidy away any work-related items, put your devices away, put on some music, light a candle or burn some essential oils in a burner', believes Salcedas.

A tidy home equals a happy mind.

This content is imported from Instagram. You may be able to find the same content in another format, or you may be able to find more information, at their web site.

Master The DIY Facial

Sticking to a strict and minimalist skincare routine has its benefits: it's simple and quick to do and you're less likely to break out if you're not trying millions of new products at once and overwhelming skin.

However, sometimes we just need a pamper or a treatment to clear up our breakouts. The best way to do this? Introduce a mask into your skincare routine to either use a couple of times a week or as a solution to use as and when you need it.

Making Your Own Spa at Home

Printed in Great Britain
by Amazon